Nutrition in a Nutshell

Kim Folsom

Writers Club Press

San Jose New York Lincoln Shanghai

Nutrition in a Nutshell

Published by Writers Club Press
an imprint of iUniverse.com, Inc.

For information address:
iUniverse.com, Inc.
620 North 48th Street
Suite 201
Lincoln, NE 68504-3467
www.iuniverse.com

ISBN: 0-595-00549-7

Printed in the United States of America

Contents

Chapter 1

Water
Hydrate Your Body

Chapter 2

To Limit, or to Eliminate?
That is the Question

Chapter 3

The Good Stuff

Chapter 4

Change is Good

Chapter 5

In a Nutshell

Acknowledgments

I would like to thank my children, Madison and Jake, and my husband, Ronnie. You three were my inspiration and motivation in writing this book. Together, we will continue our journey to healthy living. You are my greatest joys.

I must also thank my stepmother, Ann, for making homemade yogurt and never buying white bread or sugared cereal. And thank you to my mother, Joyce, for being a vegetarian and eating so much weird stuff when I was a kid. You guys were ahead of your time. I didn't know it then, but you were laying a strong foundation of nutritional wisdom that I build on every day. Thank you.

Finally, thanks to my mother, Joyce, for all the help with this book.

Introduction

Okay, so you know you could use a little help in the nutrition department. You've taken a huge step by even cracking the cover of this book, right? Lately you've heard a lot about tofu and veggie burgers and the benefits of soy. But to be perfectly honest, you've never seen tofu, you prefer your burgers with bacon, and you're not real sure what the heck soy is.

Or, maybe you've dipped your big toe in the pool of healthy eating and you're considering taking the plunge. That is, you generally order the chicken instead of the beef and you avoid fried foods. You're familiar with the food pyramid and you know you should consume five vegetables and fruits a day. You aren't a total health disaster, but you could stand a few improvements.

Welcome. You've come to the right place. I am so excited to offer a nutrition guide to average, real, everyday, ordinary people. There are plenty of books out there for tree-hugging, bark-munching vegetarian fanatics. (They're the smart ones, by the way. I aspire to be one.) But those books are intimidating and difficult to digest (pun intended). They don't really speak to everyday people like us.

I am offering this book to average people like me. I am a middle-class Mid-western mother of two. I am average amongst the average! I know how real people eat, and I know some changes are in order. I am not suggesting that you cut out all of the fun, fast, ooey-gooey, sweet, salty, cheesy, crunchy, yummy, mouth-watering treats of life. I am simply suggesting that some slight adjustments to your diet can be monumentally beneficial to your overall health. And I am offering you a place to start.

I will not nag and browbeat you about giving up all of your favorite foods. You can improve your health immensely by simply cutting back. I will, however, give you the facts on which foods are bad for you and should be limited or eliminated.

I will also give you lots of ideas for good alternatives. It's time to embrace a healthier diet.

Let me be real blunt for a moment. We as a society are fatter and more sickly than ever before. Obesity, heart disease, high blood pressure, cancer, and many other problems can be directly linked to what we eat. Our diets are loaded with fat, sugar, and chemicals. If we don't improve our diets, we're going to get sick. It's time to make some changes.

I want to help you open your eyes and your mind to the benefits of a healthier diet. I encourage you to look toward the future and possible weight or health concerns you might have. What does your family tree look like? Are there any conditions or patterns you'd like to avoid or prevent?

My family tree scares me. Three of my four grandparents have diabetes. There have been heart problems, cancer, stroke, and obesity in my family. I plan to do all I can to fortify my body and teach my children to do the same.

I was originally motivated to live a healthier life because of my children. I am solely responsible for feeding them, an awesome task to be sure. I must ensure that they are nourished, not poisoned. If you have children, it is your job to feed them well and teach them good nutritional habits.

Children are at our mercy in every way. They eat what we put in front of them. They model what they observe. This is a huge responsibility for parents. But it is also a challenge and a wonderful opportunity. We can choose to feed our children wholesome, nutritious foods. We can teach them to eat when they're **hungry** and stop when they're **comfortable**. We can promote growth, balance, and good nutritional habits that will be a way of life. What grand achievements!

After one mom spoke to me of the health benefits of the cheese in her son's cheese puff snack, I considered writing a book about nutrition. After another mom defended the fruit content in her daughter's strawberry licorice, I **committed** myself to the project. I realized some people just don't get it. The correct information is not readily available, and the marketing tactics of some food companies are downright deplorable.

I guess I should tell you I am not a physician, nutritionist, or a dietitian. This is not a medical journal and I am not a diet guru. I am a woman, a wife, a mom, a shopper, a meal planner and a cook. I have been heavy, but I'm not now. I am somewhat food-obsessed, but I want to be healthy. I want to raise healthy kids and encourage others to do the same. I sorted through a lot of material and I'm bringing you the facts.

Throughout this book, please keep one phrase in mind, "everything in moderation". You need not be intimidated or discouraged as you read. By all means, take baby steps. Ease in to health. I do not recommend going "cold turkey". That might set you up for failure.

Your goal here is to eat a healthy diet. Your plan should be to incorporate healthy choices at your own pace. Always remain open-minded. Be aware. Read labels. Pay attention to what you're putting in your mouth. And refer back to the book often for encouragement and reinforcement.

I wish you the best of luck on your journey to health. Be strong, be smart, and stick with it! Pass the information on to others. Together we can make a difference. We can help society get healthy, one person at a time!

Chapter 1

Water
Hydrate Your Body

Until fairly recently, I did not understand how very important water is to the body. But I get it now, and I want you to get it too. Water is the single most important nutrient to your body; that's why it gets it's own chapter. You are approximately 70% water. You can survive quite a while without food, but without water, you're a goner in less than a week.

Here are some important reasons your body needs water:

p.   *Regulates body temperature*

p.   *Necessary for respiration*

P.   *Necessary for digestion*

P.   *Necessary for waste removal*

P.   *Lubricates joints*

P.   *Protects and cushions vital organs*

P.   *Carries nutrients and oxygen to all cells*

P.   *Flushes out toxins*

Can you believe all the functions you need water for? It's pretty incredible. Water helps to keep your body running like a well-oiled machine. However, if you do not give your body plenty of water, part or all of these functions will suffer. Read back through the list real quick. These are all monumentally important. I know I want everything operating smoothly in my body!

I especially love the fact that water helps remove toxins from your body by literally flushing your system. Picture a bathtub after a particularly filthy child has bathed and the water has been drained. Imagine the dirt and grime and grit ringing the middle of the tub and covering the bottom. Now picture a bucket of fresh, clean water being poured in to the tub, rinsing the filth down the drain until the tub is sparkling clean. That is essentially what water does for your body. It helps to rinse away the "dirt, grime, and grit" (toxins) that build up inside of you. I can't emphasize enough…drink your water!

How much is enough?

In researching this book, I ran across a very handy way to calculate how much water you should drink each day.

1. Take your weight

2. Divide it in half

3. That number is equal to how many ounces of water you should drink each day

For example:150 pounds divided in half=75
75 ounces of water=about 9 glasses (8 oz)

If you try that formula and you're floating away, you can always go back to the good old "6 to 8 glasses a day" theory. In most cases, that will be sufficient. However, if you lead a particularly active lifestyle and sweat a lot, you'll require more. Remember, we're talking about **water** here. All other drinks are "extras". Caffeinated beverages don't count. Don't even count non-caffeinated beverages if you can avoid it. Your body needs clean, clear water.

As long as I mentioned clean, clear water, I may as well take the opportunity to talk about the *quality* of the water you drink. It is very important for you to drink "good" water. Drinking water is one of the major sources of environmental toxins. And I hate to tell you, but the water from your tap is probably not safe. Laws regarding water are inadequate and enforcement is weak. Regulated "safe" levels of contaminants are way too high.

In short, if your drinking water isn't making you sick now, it probably will eventually. It could contain high levels of chlorine, arsenic, radon, nitrates, viruses, parasites, micro-organisms, pesticides, and herbicides. Yummy! Make no mistake, the levels of these contaminants allowed to be in "safe" drinking water are not levels you would approve of. And they can cause cancer and many other health problems.

What can you do? Drink purified water. If you can afford to, install a purification system in your home. Or, you can use a filtration pitcher. At the very least, buy water from a source you know is safe. I am convinced that a "reverse osmosis" system with a carbon filter is the best choice right now for purifying water. I have a Reverse Osmosis (RO) system under my kitchen sink. The purified water is dispensed at the sink and runs to the ice maker in my freezer...don't put contaminated ice cubes in pure water!

If you want to begin by having your water tested, use an independent lab, not a company trying to sell you their products. Then do a little research and decide what will work best for you. Most large grocery stores have pure water or RO systems and allow you to fill your own jugs fairly cheaply. If you purchase a system for your home, always keep good maintenance habits. Dirty filters can be dangerous.

Please note that bottled and purified water probably do not contain fluoride. You may need a fluoride supplement. Most adults will get enough from a fluoride tooth paste. Children may require extra. Check with your dentist or pediatrician.

One last word on contaminated water: beware of bottled water. At this time, bottled water is not regulated. You have no proof that what you're drinking is safe, unless you are sure about the source. Anybody can bottle water, slap a label on it, and sell it. Better that you know first hand how your water is purified.

Dehydration

In case you're not convinced about the importance of water, let's discuss what happens when your body doesn't get enough.

First of all, you should not wait until you're thirsty to drink. If you feet thirsty, you're probably already dehydrated, if only slightly. You should drink water consistently throughout the day.

Caffeinated beverages are not good for you and should be limited. Caffeine acts as a diuretic, which means it causes your body to discharge urine. That can cause dehydration. It is a good idea to counter each caffeinated beverage with an extra glass of water.

Here are some problems associated with dehydration:

* Dark circles under your eyes

* Headache

* Nausea

* Vomiting

* Heart burn

* Joint pain

* Hypertension

* Fatigue

* Constipation

  …just to name a few.

Headache is a particularly common symptom of dehydration that is often overlooked. Many times I have had a nagging headache and cured it with water. Sound strange? Give it a try. The next time you feel a headache coming on, try to recall how much water you've consumed that day. If you haven't had much, or any, try drinking two or three glasses over the course of an hour or so.

Then continue drinking water throughout the rest of the day. Hydrating your body can do wonders!

If you have children, it is particularly important that you pay attention to their water consumption each day. Too often, children are given sugary drinks throughout the day. Take time to read the labels of the drinks you are giving your kids. Are the juice boxes 100% real juice? If the ingredients are sugar, sucrose, high fructose corn syrup, etc…, these are not healthy drinks. Carbonated beverages are not good either.

Sugary drinks should be eliminated or limited. They aren't good hydrators because the body actually loses liquid trying to digest the sugar. And carbonated beverages pack a one-two punch with sugar and phosphoric acid. Phosphoric acid is hard on the stomach and robs the body of essential minerals. Water is what the body needs! Use the previously mentioned formula to calculate the amount of water children need, too. Remember, children are often very active and can dehydrate quickly.

A friend of mine brought her daughter over one afternoon to play with my daughter. It was a warm, sunny afternoon and the kids were playing outside. After a while, the little girl came in and told me she had a headache and didn't feel well. Her cheeks were flushed, and she felt warm to the touch. She was crying and suddenly started vomiting. Her mother picked her up and took her home, where she slept all afternoon. Sounds like the flu, huh? Well, apparently this was a pattern, so my friend took her daughter to the doctor. The child was suffering from dehydration. She was not consuming adequate amounts of water throughout the day and her body was responding with this pattern of headache, vomiting, and drowsiness. My friend began sending a bottle of water to school with her daughter and monitoring her intake of water at home. Guess what? Problem solved.

Incidentally, in case you're judging, my friend is not a neglectful mother. She's a wonderful mother and quite intelligent. This can happen to anyone. And it is more common than you would imagine. I simply wanted to illustrate my point. Everyone must drink plenty of water!

So there you have it, the low-down on water. It's pretty clear cut. Your body absolutely needs plenty of water every day in order to operate properly. Give your body what it needs!

Chapter 2

To Limit, or to Eliminate?
That is the Question

Welcome to the nasty chapter of this book. I figure I may as well get this part over early and then I'll move on to the good stuff. In this chapter, I'll tell you which foods and additives may be bad for you and why. I'll keep it simple and to the point, without using a lot of dull scientific gibberish. I weeded through the scientific gibberish so that I could give it to you in plain English. As you read, don't be discouraged. There are plenty of other good foods out there and I'm going to help you find them. And remember, "everything in moderation". You do not have to give up everything in this chapter. I am suggesting that you start by limiting these foods, and go from there. I am not the boss of you! You are the boss of you! So, you'll decide what to give up and when.

Partially Hydrogenated Oil

I decided to begin this chapter with partially hydrogenated (hi-draw-jenated) oil because it gets very little attention, but is quite dangerous. I'm sure most of you don't have a clue as to what it is or why it's bad. Unlike sugar and some of the other "bad guys", partially hydrogenated oil doesn't get much press. I think it's high time to change that.

To *hydrogenate* is to combine with hydrogen, or to reduce with hydrogen. Basically, hydrogen is added to oils to make them solid and to prolong their shelf life. This process creates trans fatty acids (TFAs), which you probably have heard of. TFAs have been proven to increase the incidence of cancer and are associated with increased risk of heart disease.

Basically, the trans fatty acid is a man-made, synthetic molecule that gets in to our cells, interrupting optimum function. Our bodies do not recognize the TFAs and can not utilize or remove them. They damage our cells, causing a decline in our immune system. And the damage is cumulative, meaning it will build up over time as long as we consume hydrogenated oils.

This is truly one of the scariest health hazards because people aren't aware of the danger. It has been predicted that the accumulating evidence about the detrimental effects of partially hydrogenated oils will force them to be banned from foods in the near future. Until then, you must protect yourself. And if you're like I used to be, you tell yourself, "It can't be that bad or it wouldn't be on the shelves"...wake up! You have to protect yourself, because when there is big money involved, as with the food companies, your protection is not a big concern. They won't make any changes until enough people make enough noise and they are forced to make changes.

Where will you find partially hydrogenated oil? Brace yourself, it's everywhere! The obvious culprits are solid vegetable shortenings (Crisco), and margarine. My advice to you is throw these away immediately and replace them in your cooking. They are very unhealthy. The next place to look is at snack foods. Really, almost all of the packaged food you buy contains partially hydrogenated oil. Start reading the labels of your favorite chips, cookies, snack crackers, cereals, and peanut butter. Even that loaf of bread in your kitchen probably contains partially hydrogenated oil. But that's not all. The next time you're eating out and you order those french fries, consider the fact that most restaurants use partially hydrogenated oil to fry food. Remember, it prolongs the shelf life of food because it doesn't get rancid as quickly as natural oil. That is why food companies use it. That is also why you can have that box of crackers in your pantry for six months or more! But at what cost to your health?

With the exception of solid shortening and margarine, I recommend you begin to limit the amount of partially hydrogenated oil you consume. I recommend you immediately and completely stop using shortening and margarine. You are definitely better off using real dairy butter (moderately). At least it is a natural, not synthetic substance. Also, you can begin experimenting with some of the alternatives I give you later in the book. Again, don't be discouraged. I promise there are plenty of good snack foods that don't contain partially hydrogenated oil, and many of them taste the same, if not better! Of course, ideally you will eliminate partially hydrogenated oil from your diet completely, But start by cutting back. I can't stress strongly enough, this stuff is dangerous.

Artificial Sweeteners

I am putting artificial sweeteners right behind partially hydrogenated oil because I think it is another dangerous substance that people just don't know enough about.

I would like to emphasize one point; if you have children, never allow them to consume artificial sweeteners in any form. Never, never, never. They were never intended for general public consumption, they are not natural, and they are poison to our bodies. Children have died from consumption of artificial sweeteners. People have had terrible health problems related to the use of artificial sweeteners and some are suffering now and don't know the cause. This is one subject which has no gray area. Get artificial sweeteners out of your diet!

Aspartame

Aspartame is made by the Sherwin Williams Paint Company from petroleum products. It is a non-food product. It is marketed under the names NutraSweet and Equal. Aspartame consists of three chemicals; aspartic acid, phenylalanine, and methanol. These *chemicals* are not recognizable to the body. When consumed, these *chemicals* are released in to the blood stream.

HELLO !?!
Did you notice the word CHEMICALS?

Problems linked to Aspartame consumption:

P.   *Dizziness*

P.   *Headache*

P.   *Visual impairment*

P.   *Disorientation*

P.   *Muscle aches*

P.   *Numbing of extremities*

P. *High blood pressure*

P. *Inflammation of the pancreas*

P. *Hemorrhaging of the eyes*

P. *Sleeping problems*

P. *Thyroid problems*

P. *Memory loss*

P. *Graves disease*

According to research, chemicals in Aspartame pose a significant threat to the developing nervous systems of fetuses, infants, and young children.

It has been cited that consumption of Aspartame during pregnancy may adversely affect brain function in developing fetuses.

Chemicals in Aspartame are toxic to the brain in high concentrations.

So, is saccharin better? Heck no! Saccharin has been proven to cause cancer in test animals. It is completely banned in Canada (and should be in this country). Why do you think the law requires *warning labels* about saccharin on food packages? It's very dangerous!

Let me make this very clear. Artificial sweeteners are unnatural, unhealthy, and hazardous to your body. You should not consume them in any form. They are found in diet sodas, cookies, diet foods, candy, and even gum. Read labels! Pay attention! You may feel fine now, but how do you know that these chemicals aren't wreaking havoc in your body? Do you want to find out the hard way? Don't take a chance with your health. Avoid artificial sweeteners completely.

Saturated Fat

Fat has been in the limelight for a long time. I remember when I went on my "low fat" diet. I counted fat grams, not paying attention to anything else. I hate to think of the amounts of sugar and other calories I consumed. But I counted those fat grams! Did I lose weight? Oh yeah. And hair. Yep, my hair started to fall out. And my fingernails were paper-thin and layered like flintstone. And my skin was dry and flaky. What a mess! The truth is, your body needs a certain amount of fat in order to function properly.

I urge you to avoid the "low fat" trap. Many "low fat" snacks are loaded with sugar and other junk. And frankly, you should be more worried about sugar and other toxins. Do not attempt to eliminate fat from your diet. You just need to pay attention to the type of fat you consume and the amount. Your intake of saturated fat should definitely be limited.

What is saturated fat? Basically, it is any form of animal fat. Meat, poultry, dairy, and eggs all contain saturated fat. A few others include coconut oil, chocolate, and anything made with lard. Saturated fat is the least healthy fat because it is highest in cholesterol. High cholesterol is linked to heart disease and cancer.

So you must begin to limit your consumption of saturated fat. Optimally, you would not consume any animal products, thereby avoiding the whole problem. But, realistically, if you will pay attention to your diet and cut back on animal products, coconut oil, and chocolate, you'll be on the right track.

Sugar

If you were going to completely eliminate any one thing from your diet, your best choice would probably be sugar. I know, you have a sweet tooth. Me, too. I'm just telling you the stuff is bad for you. It is disruptive to your whole system and should definitely be limited. The damage done by sugar can manifest itself in many health problems. Some of those problems are: diabetes, hypoglycemia, osteoporosis, heart disease, cancer, arthritis, obesity, asthma, and tooth decay. Other, less serious problems are: headaches, constipation, and gas.

Here's the Scoop

- Sugar is laden with toxins

- Sugar suppresses the immune system

- Sugar impairs the body's ability to fight off disease

- Sugar disrupts digestion

- Eating sugar keeps the body's enzymes and minerals constantly out of balance

- Sugar interferes with the body's ability to absorb and utilize minerals

- Sugar consumption has been directly linked to calcium depletion

- Sugar completely disrupts your body chemistry

Enough said. I think you get my point. So, what should you do? Pay attention! Read labels! Watch out for hidden sugar. Sucrose, fructose, and corn syrup are all sugars. Start by regulating the amount of sugar you add to your food at home. Then begin to read the labels on foods before you buy them or eat them. When you begin to pay attention to your diet, you will be amazed by the amount of sugar you have been consuming. The average American eats over 100 pounds of sugar each year!

Refined white sugar is chemically processed in such a way that it is stripped of all nutrients and full of toxins. Other chemically processed sugars include, brown sugar, raw sugar, and corn syrup. All of these should be limited. They provide empty calories (no nutrients) and are all detrimental to the body.

If you have children, by all means monitor their intake of sugar. Snack foods, drinks, cereals, candy and gum marketed to children are full of sugar. Their little bodies can not tolerate being inundated by sugar. It damages their immune systems, leaving them more susceptible to illness. Plus, if their tummies are being filled up with sugary snacks and drinks, they probably aren't getting enough of the healthy, nutritious foods they need for optimum growth and function.

Basically, sugar is not good for any of us, we all eat too much, and we all need to cut back.

Meat

I am mostly talking about red meat here (beef, pork, and lamb) but I will briefly discuss poultry at the end of this section.

This is a sticky subject for me to speak about. Remember I told you I live in the Midwest? Well, I live near Kansas City, Missouri. This is truly a "cow town". People around here raise cattle and they take their steaks and bar-b-que very seriously. I grew up on Kansas City strip steaks and Gates Bar-B-Que! But I don't eat any of that any more. I decided to give up red meat.

Why? Well, I did some research. I sought out books, articles, and studies on red meat. I was overwhelmingly convinced that it just isn't very healthy. I could go on and on about the inhumane treatment of the animals and the conditions at slaughter houses, because it is very disturbing. But, I want to focus on what makes red meat unhealthy.

Don't have a cow!

Protein

Meat contains concentrated protein. Excess protein has been linked to kidney stones, osteoporosis, heart disease, and cancer. Animal proteins tend to deplete calcium, which can lead to osteoporosis.

Fat and Cholesterol

Meat is loaded with fat and cholesterol. Fat and cholesterol are known causes of heart disease.

Hormones

Farmers have to compete. They must feed the cows and other livestock growth hormones so they'll grow real big, real fast. Not only can the hormones be found in the flesh of the animals, they're concentrated. When we consume animal products, we consume growth hormones.

Antibiotics

Livestock raised for consumption in this country are unhealthy. They are fed antibiotics to fight off infection and disease. 55% of all antibiotics in the U.S. are fed to livestock. Bacteria are becoming resistant and even immune to these antibiotics. We consume the flesh of these animals. Our bodies are becoming resistant to antibiotics.

Pesticides

Fields are treated with pesticides. The livestock graze on or are fed from the fields, they consume the pesticides, which are concentrated in their flesh. Meat contains dangerously high quantities of pesticide residues.

___Digestion___

Meat is difficult for your body to digest. It taxes your system and can zap your energy.

___Cancer___

People who regularly eat meat, especially red meat, are more likely to get cancer.

At this point, you're probably imagining that life without red meat is an option. You'll just eat more chicken, right? I'm not so sure that's the answer. There are definite problems with poultry, too. Chicken farmers, like all farmers, are in the business to make a living. They must compete. Chickens are also fed growth hormones and antibiotics. Plus, they are often raised and slaughtered in filthy, disgusting conditions. Much of the chicken raised for human consumption is contaminated with Salmonella and other bacteria.

Now what? Don't be discouraged. "Free-range" chicken products are more widely available now than ever before. Free-range chickens are allowed to roam and grow naturally with no hormones. They are fed a healthy, natural diet without antibiotics mixed in. They are also slaughtered in more sanitary, humane conditions. Free-range chicken can still be a bit difficult to find and is, or course, more expensive. But if you search it out, and cut back on the red meat you buy, you can probably swing it. You may have to ask your grocer to get it for you. Just do your best to make sure it is **certified** range-free. The extra time, effort, and money will be well worth it.

Dairy Products

Now, before you come unglued, here me out. I used to be a big proponent of milk and other dairy products. I drank milk all the time, not just because I thought it was good for me, but because I loved it! But, through research and experimentation, I've changed my mind. Dairy cows are not healthy like they once were. They are diseased and their udders are so over-stimulated that they develop ulcers called mastitis, which are treated with antibiotics. So, pus from the infections **and** antibiotics are in the milk. Pasteurization is intended to kill bacteria in milk, not remove pus , antibiotics, pesticides, or steroids. The cows are often given feed which has been treated with pesticides. And they are injected with steroids to enhance milk production. An average dairy cow will produce up to fifty quarts of milk a day, up from nine quarts a day in 1960. And all of this junk from the cows' bodies are passed on in their milk.

If that's not enough to gross you out, consider this: dairy products are loaded with fat and cholesterol, which have been linked to heart disease, kidney stones, arthritis, depression, diabetes, cancer, and allergies. At least fifty per cent of all American children are allergic to milk, and at least that many adults are lactose intolerant. (Lactose is found in milk and is difficult for some people to digest.) Dairy products are the leading cause of allergies in this country. They are also mucus-forming and therefore worsen conditions such as asthma and sinus infection.

The bottom line is, humans were intended to consume human milk, and only during infancy. How many adults do you know that drink breast milk? Cow's milk is designed to nourish a calf and turn it in to a cow. Cows don't drink milk, only calves do. We are the only species that drinks milk in adulthood. And, we're the only species that drinks the milk of another animal. Think of any other animal in the entire animal kingdom. Would you drink elephant milk? Pig milk? How about ice cream made from monkey milk? It's really pretty disgusting when you think of it like that.

When I decided to try eliminating dairy products, I did it for health reasons. As a bonus, I lost seven pounds in two weeks! My stomach felt better and my skin looked better. It was great! The truth is, since I gave up meat and cut back on dairy, I have been able to easily maintain my weight, I no longer eat antacids like candy, and I haven't had a migraine headache in a very long time. (I don't know specifically what made the migraine headaches go away, because I now eat a much healthier diet and have removed a lot of the toxins I used to regularly consume.) When I started, I stayed completely off dairy, very strictly, for several months. Now I would say I stay away from dairy. Occasionally I fall off the wagon completely, but I usually limit it carefully. Also, I buy mostly organic dairy products.

I'm sure you're feeling a little confused because of all of the good things you've always heard about milk. And you're probably wondering how you will get enough calcium if you limit or eliminate dairy products. For all of the reasons I have mentioned, and many more, milk is just not as healthy as the dairy counsel would like you to believe. Remember, when there is big money involved, you must educate and protect yourself. The truth is, there are many sources of calcium that are much healthier. (See chapter four.)

I have discussed eliminating dairy products with many people. Some people are more receptive than others. Limiting or eliminating dairy helped my son's seasonal allergies, my niece's diaper rash, and a friend's constant stuffiness. Removing dairy from your diet can help you lose weight, clear up skin problems, and improve allergy symptoms as well as stomach problems. I can't imagine that a parent with an allergic child wouldn't give it a shot. At the very least, I recommend limiting dairy products for over-all better health. There are many good alternatives and better sources of calcium. You must simply be open-minded and willing to try new things.

When my little niece was a tiny infant, she had terrible diaper rash. My brother and sister-in law changed her diaper constantly, let her bottom air out often, and kept her very clean and dry. But the rash persisted. They made several trips to the pediatrician, who finally concluded that the baby might be allergic to dairy products. My sister-in law was nursing, so that meant she would have to give up dairy to see if the rash cleared up. As luck would have it, I had been dairy-free for several months, so I educated my sister-in law on the wonders of dairy substitutes! My brother committed to eliminating dairy as well, to be supportive. Two weeks later, the rash was gone! And it never returned. That was nearly a year ago and they are all still dairy-free and doing great!

Even if you don't have allergies, a weight problem, or any health conditions that you're worried about now, I would suggest cutting back on dairy. Everyone I know who has tried it just feels better.

Food Additives

Chemicals, Artificial Colorings, Artificial Flavorings, Preservatives

Chemicals are man-made. They do not occur naturally, therefore they are not favorable to your body. Excessive exposure to chemicals inside your body can lead to toxic poisoning, which can manifest itself in many ways, including cancer. Toxic poisoning can cause organ dysfunction and a weakened immune system.

You would be shocked to know the huge amounts of chemicals you consume. Food additives can be found in most packaged and processed foods. They are added to enhance flavor and color, and to prolong shelf life. That's great for the manufacturers and retailers. It's not so great for you. In fact, food additives actually poison your body. You may not feel any symptoms of chemical poisoning now, but the damage can be cumulative. That means the toxins may be building up in your body and may not cause problems for a long time. Are you willing to gamble with your health?

The only way to rid your body of this potential poisoning is to begin to remove packaged, processed foods from your diet. The more **fresh** food you eat, the healthier you will be. When your body is no longer over-taxed with chemicals, it will be better equipped to keep you strong and healthy. Your immune system will improve and you'll have more energy.

Artificial Colorings

These are used to enhance the appearance of food. Most are synthetic, meaning man-made (not natural). They have no nutritional value. Many have been linked to cancer and other health concerns.

MSG

(Monosodium Glutamate)

This is a substance added to food to enhance flavor. It's also used as a preservative. It's often prevalent in Chinese food. Many people are highly allergic to MSG. Some people are sensitive to it and don't know it. Watch for the words "hydrolyzed" and "autolyzed yeast" which always refer to MSG. MSG can be disguised, so check the labels of processed foods. Look for the terms "textured vegetable protein (TVP) or plant protein extract. Some symptoms of MSG are headache, swelling and chest tightness.

Nitrites and Nitrates

These are the chemical preservatives used to cure processed meat such as lunchmeat and hot-dogs. These preservatives have been linked to cancer in humans.

Sodium

Salt. Sodium is used to enhance flavor and preserve foods, often in large amounts. Salt consumption has been linked to high blood pressure. Watch for sodium content in packaged foods. It is often grossly over used.

Children and Food Additives

Regarding children, studies have shown that food additives can interrupt brain function. They can cause drowsiness, stimulation, and headaches. In extreme cases, food additives have been linked to severe behavioral and attention disorders. Because children are small, and we tend to feed them a lot of packaged and processed food, they often have especially strong reactions to the chemicals. The awful part is, we usually don't link the reactions to the source.

Basically, if you've never heard of it or you can't pronounce it, avoid it. If you pick up a package of food and the label is as long as your arm, avoid it. If the ingredients include "artificial" anything, avoid it. Stop saturating your body with chemical-laden food. Here's an idea…try some fresh food!

Pesticides

Pesticides are very difficult to avoid. Unfortunately, they are widely used and most are deemed acceptable by the FDA. However, I'm sure that if we, the general public, were educated about pesticides, we would flatly refuse them in our food.

They are very bad for human consumption.

Pesticides are used to kill pests (obviously) and preserve crops. They are used on vegetables, fruits, and grains. They are also used on the crops which are harvested to feed the livestock we consume. Furthermore, pesticide residues saturate the fields that are treated, and run off in to our streams, contaminating our water sources. Consumption of pesticides has been linked to illnesses such as cancer.

To avoid consuming pesticides, you can seek out foods which are "certified organic". According to the California Organic Foods Act of 1990, foods can only be labeled "certified organic" if they are grown and processed organically, with no chemical pesticides.

If organic food is difficult to find in your area, there are other precautions you can take. Wash your fruits and vegetables thoroughly with a mild soap that is made especially for washing produce, then rinse well. Or you can buy products that you spray on to remove wax and pesticides. These products can usually be found in the produce department of your grocery store. Also, it's a good idea to peel fruits and vegetables when you can.

Chapter 3

The Good Stuff

Now it's time to talk about what you **can** and **should** eat. I'm so excited to share this information with you. I sincerely hope you will give it a chance. Forget about any prejudice you may have toward healthy food. Do you think only junk food tastes good? That is so wrong. Healthy food can taste great and since it is so vitally important to your best health, please keep an open mind. These foods should make up the bulk of your diet. If you ate only these foods, prepared in a healthy manner, you'd be a picture of health. However, I understand that you are very busy and "convenience food" is just so, well, convenient. I'm just suggesting that you start adding more of this "real food" in to you diet.

In 1991, the Physicians Committee for Responsible Medicine recommended a new food pyramid, consisting of four new food groups. They suggested that the current four food groups (meat, dairy, grains, fruits and vegetables), be replaced by: grains, legumes, vegetables, fruit. The committee reported that we should consume a plant-based diet for optimum health.

The current four food groups have been part of the US government recommendations since 1956. This food pyramid, with meat as the base, or the largest group, may be largely responsible for declining health and serious illness such as heart disease, cancer and stroke.

By adjusting your diet to include more of the "new four food groups" and less meat and dairy, you will be eliminating a great deal of saturated fat and cholesterol. That adjustment will improve your health immensely and help protect you from illness and disease.

Whole Grains

The term "whole grain" is pretty self-explanatory, but let me give you a quick run down on the benefits of eating whole grain food. First of all, a grain seed is made up of three basic parts, the germ (the seed), the endosperm (starch), and the bran (the outer shell). Each part is nutritionally beneficial, and together they contain almost every nutrient your body needs. Whole grains provide carbohydrate energy and are a good source of protein and fiber, but only when you consume the *whole grain.*

That brings me to the problem with white bread and anything made with white flour. During the commercial refining process of wheat, the germ and the bran are removed, leaving only the endosperm (starch). The endosperm has less food value than the other two parts. A long time ago it was discovered that the germ of the wheat was the part that sprouted and caused the flour to spoil. The germ was also the part that the rodents and insects would go for (smart critters). So began the process of degerming. Removing the bran, as well, left a more aesthetic, smoother, whiter, prettier flour. White flour became preferred, whole wheat flour became obsolete. Nutritionally superior flour was replaced by a fluffy, processed substance almost devoid of any nutritional value.

What about the "enriched" flours and breads? Well, the manufacturers do attempt to replace some of the vitamins and minerals with synthetic replacements. But the man-made impostor nutrients aren't as body-friendly as the real things. And, only *some* of the vitamins and minerals are replaced. In addition, products made with white flour often contain: preservatives, partially hydrogenated oil, artificial flavorings, artificial colorings, dough conditioners, mold inhibitors, and huge amounts of salt and sugars (in various forms). Don't forget about the bleaching process, which makes the bread that pristine white and keeps the insects out. That is done with *chemicals* such as chlorine dioxide. (At what point in history did human beings lose their minds?) There are more than eighty additives that may legally be added to bread. Yum!

The answer to chemical-laden, nutritionally defunct bread is *whole grain* bread. Specifically, the package must read, "100% whole wheat", or the first ingredient should be "whole wheat flour". Not "enriched", not "bleached". You have to be careful here, because many breads *appear* to be very healthy. Clever packaging and a catchy name can fool the best of us. Read the label before you buy the product. This will ensure you're getting the benefits of the *whole grain.*

Furthermore, selecting other whole grain products is important. Whole wheat pasta and brown rice are good examples. Whole wheat pasta is made with the whole grain and brown rice has it's nutritional bran coat still intact. (White rice is what is left when the bran coat is removed.) It is lighter and fluffier, but is stripped of most of it's vital nutrients.

Whole grain foods are nutritionally superior to their processed counterparts and are an important part of a well-balanced diet. The type of fiber in whole grains is responsible for absorbing water in your digestive tract, which helps soften your stools, making them pass easily. It also helps to clean out your colon. (Believe me, I don't want to discuss this any more than you do, but it's **important**! Colon cancer is a very serious problem in this country and this is one thing you can do to protect yourself.) Go for the grains!

Legumes

Beans
Soy Beans and all Soy products
Peas
Peanuts

All of the above are legumes. They grow in the ground and are loaded with good nutrition. All legumes provide an excellent source of vegetable protein. Vegetable protein is easier to digest that animal protein, therefore it is less taxing to your system. Legumes are also a good source of fiber, iron, calcium, zinc and B vitamins.

Soy What?

What is the big deal about soy? Well, soy is one of the most nutritious sources of plant protein. It's a complete protein, which means it's balanced in all essential amino acids. It offers many health bene-fits and can completely replace animal protein without the risky side affects. However, if you do not wish to give up meat, adding soy to your diet can greatly improve your health.

What the heck is it?

- All soy products are made from soy beans
- Some examples of soy products are: tofu (I know you've heard of it), tempeh (what?), miso (huh?), soy nuts, soy milk, soy cheese, soy burgers, soy hot dogs, soy ice cream...see chapter 4!

What are the health benefits?

Most importantly, soy beans contain isoflavones, which are naturally occurring plant nutrients. These nutrients include Phytoestrogens and Antioxidants.

Phytoestrogen Benefits

- Phytoestrogens help to regulate hormone levels in both men and women
- Studies have shown soy consumption helps reduce symptoms of menopause *without* hormone replacement drugs
- Soy consumption may help reduce the occurrence of hormone-dependent cancers such as

> breast cancer, prostate cancer, ovarian cancer and uterine cancer

- Soy consumption may also help reduce the occurrence of conditions such as fibrocystic changes in breasts, uterine fibroids, and endometriosis.

Antioxidant Benefits

First of all, **antioxidants** are vitamins in foods or supplements which boost the immune system by repairing damage done by **free radicals**.

Free radicals are molecules which are created by toxins in your body. They cause health problems by damaging healthy cells and tissues.

Cancer occurs when cells are damaged and multiply, crowding out healthy cells.

- Therefore, soy consumption may reduce the occurrence of cancer.

As if that weren't enough...

- Other components of soy have been found to lower cholesterol levels, which reduces the risk of heart disease.

- Consumption of soy may help battle calcium depletion and osteoporosis.

Although I have mostly discussed soy beans, all legumes are very healthy. I concentrated on soy because I'm convinced that you just don't have the facts. To most of you, tofu seems weird, and soy products are foreign. I'm hoping to change that.

Vegetables

Five servings of vegetables and fruits **each day** are recommended as part of a healthy diet. You should make it **mandatory** for yourself and any-one you are responsible for feeding. By the way, that means five servings of vegetables and fruits combined (such as, three servings of vegetables and two servings of fruits), or any combination you desire.

Regarding vegetables, eat **fresh** vegetables when-ever possible. Choose frozen as your next option, and canned as your last choice. Canned vegeta-bles are generally over-cooked, which depletes their nutritional value. Also, they often contain huge amounts of sodium and other additives.

Vegetables are a great source of many vitamins and minerals. They offer antioxidant (disease fighting) protection and are an important source of fiber. Dietary fiber helps you avoid "elimination problems" such as constipation and diarrhea.

You should eat a variety of vegetables in all colors as they each contain unique nutrients. Your vegetable intake should include green, red, orange, and yellow selections. However, you have to be careful about a few: corn, peas, and potatoes are all very starchy or sugary vegetables. When you eat these they convert to sugar in your body. I'm not saying they're **bad** for you. You just have to consider them a "starch" and still get plenty of what I would call "better" vegetables. Eating a good *variety* of veggies is the key.

Eat your vegetables! They're good for you!

Fruit

Fruit can be considered the great cleanser. The type of fiber in fruit (soluble fiber) collects and carries bad cholesterol (LDL) and other toxins through your system so they can be eliminated. Fruit is essential to keeping your system operating smoothly.

Fruit is loaded with important vitamins and minerals, some of which are in short supply from any other food group. Just as with vegetables, you should eat a variety of fruits and choose fresh selections when you can. Frozen fruits are next best, canned are the least nutritionally beneficial.

It is important to remember that fruit is full of sugar. Even though it's natural sugar, you still have to consider it in your daily intake of sugars. Some people are more sensitive to sugars and carbohydrates than others. If you don't have a weight problem or blood sugar problems, you don't have to worry as much.

Have some fruit every day!

Chapter 4

Change is Good

Let's begin this chapter by taking a deep breath and exhaling slowly. I have given you a lot of information and I know it can be overwhelming. However, as I said in the introduction, "everything in moderation". Do not allow yourself to be intimidated or discouraged. Take baby steps.

You need not go from junk food junkie to barkmuncher overnight. I would suggest that you begin by simply paying attention to what you're buying, preparing, eating, and serving your family. You have to stop aimlessly putting everything in your mouth and take time to think about what you're eating. If you're responsible for feeding children, you should be extra careful. Start reading labels at the grocery store. If a food label is full of nutritional no-no's, don't buy it. Or, make a conscious effort to limit the no-no's and replace them with better choices **most** of the time. You must begin to pay attention and read labels.

I challenge you to go to your kitchen and begin reading labels. How many items list sugar or a form of sugar as one of the first few ingredients? How many labels list partially hydrogenated oil? Do you have solid shortening such as Crisco in your cabinet? Do you use margarine?

You must become a militant label reader. In the beginning it may be a pain in the neck, but as you get used to **paying attention**, you'll find it will become a habit. Any time I consider buying an unfamiliar package of food, I pick it up, flip it over, and check for unhealthy ingredients. Train yourself to do the same.

Now, lets discuss your new diet...

First of all, you aren't "going on a diet". I'm not going to tell you exactly how to eat, meal by meal. Your new diet is simply going to include healthier choices. You should start limiting and eliminating the junk at your own pace. Don't put so much pressure on yourself that you'll get discouraged and fail. Failure means going back to eating too much junk and that's not acceptable. If you slip up, don't give up. Just give yourself a break and start all over. Remember, the goals are better health, more energy, and less illness. It is so worth the effort!

Focus on eating more natural foods and less processed foods. Food is healthiest right from the source. The more removed from the source it is, the less nutritional value it has. That is why processed, over-cooked, chemical-laden packaged food is not good for you.

Have you heard the term "shop the walls"? This is a great rule to follow. By shopping the walls of your grocery store, you'll buy from the produce, frozen, dairy, and meat sections. This is where you'll find the most nutritious selections. (In the dairy and meat section, go organic if possible.) The further in to the interior of the store you go, the more processed, packaged junk food you'll find. Shop the walls!

Foods to Limit or Eliminate
(and why)

Drinks

soft drinks: too much sugar, phosphoric acid

sugary drinks: teas, juice cocktails, kool-aid, most kid drinks

diet drinks: artificial sweeteners

hot chocolate: too much sugar

cappuccino: mixes and machine versions may contain partially hydrogenated oil far too much fat and sugar

Breakfast

sugary cereals: empty calories

doughnuts, cinnamon rolls, etc.: refined flour, refined sugar, empty calories

prepared or boxed breakfasts: additives, sugar, partially hydrogenated oil

toaster pastries: too much sugar, partially hydrogenated oil, empty calories

cereal bars: same junk as toaster pastries

breakfast meats (bacon, sausage, etc.): saturated fat, too much sodium, additives

flavored oatmeal: too much sugar

frozen pancakes/waffles: refined flour, too much sugar, partially hydrogenated oil

Pancake mixes: partially hydrogenated oil, additives

fast food restaurant breakfast: too much saturated fat, partially hydrogenated oil, additives, sugar

Lunch

packaged lunch meat: preservatives and additives such as nitrites and nitrates

hot dogs: same as lunch meat

white bread: refined flour, little nutrients, no fiber

process cheese food, prepared cheese product (Velveeta and other packaged cheese): overly processed

pre-packaged lunches (such as Lunchables): high fat content, additives, sugary drinks

frozen meals: partially hydrogenated oil, high fat content, preservatives and other additives

canned lunches (such as pastas, etc.): over-processed, little nutritional value, additives

fried foods: saturated fat, partially hydro-genated oil

fast food: too much of all the bad stuff

Dinner

dinners from a box (Helpers): additives, partially hydrogenated oil, little little nutritional value

frozen meals: see lunches

fried foods: see lunches

fast foods: see lunches

Examples of Healthier Choices

Drinks

water

tea, especially herb tea

coffee, preferably decaffeinated

natural fruit juice

soy drinks

rice drinks

Breakfast

fruit

whole grain toast, whole grain muffins, whole grain bagels

eggs (whites only if cholesterol is a problem)

whole grain cereals

vegetarian meat alternatives

Lunch

natural peanut butter w/ natural fruit spread

whole grain breads

homemade tuna salad

lean, fresh deli meats

beans

canned soup (make healthy selections, check labels for too much salt, etc.)

salads w/ healthy dressings (check labels for additives)

vegetables

Dinner

grilled or baked fish

grilled or baked chicken (organic if possible)

lean cuts of meat in small portions (organic if possible)

beans

vegetables-steamed, baked, roasted

whole grain brown rice

whole wheat pasta

Making the Changes

First of all, you need to add the words "health food store" to your vocabulary. If there is not one near you, go to the largest grocery store near you or ask your grocer to carry some of the items you can't find.

The only big, full-line health food store near me is about 40 minutes away. I shop there when I can, but I rely heavily on my grocery store. Also, there is a really good, smaller health food store about 15 minutes from my home. They carry a good selection so I shop there often.

I find many healthier choices at the two large chain grocery stores I frequent. At first, I had to scan the aisles carefully, but now I know where the healthy treasures are kept.

In the beginning, you may have to do a little research. Check your phone book under "health" to locate a store in your area. If you live in a rural or remote area, it may be more of a challenge to find a health food store. But you will probably do well if you can at least find a large, full-line grocery store.

I know that some of the health food choices can be quite expensive. This can be discouraging. I have had a very limited grocery budget in the past and just did my best to select more fresh food and less processed food.

You will find that as you begin to choose healthier foods on a regular basis, you will be eliminating a lot of unnecessary junk food that can really add up. Sugary drinks, sugary cereals, chips, snack cakes and other packaged foods can really be expensive. Just remember that you are making an investment in your health. With your particular budget in mind, choose the healthiest food you can afford.

The most important thing to remember when choosing a healthier diet is that you must be **OPEN MINDED**.

Soy milk and rice milk **are not cow's milk**. So do not expect them to taste like the milk you're used to. View them as a *new* taste. Also, cheeses, ice creams, and other derivatives of these milks will not taste exactly like the dairy products you're used to.

With that in mind, I can promise you that if you give them a chance, many of these new, healthier foods will surprise you. Be willing to sample different flavors and different brands to discover your favorites. And never lose sight of the goal...better health.

A suggestion would be to begin by having one vegetarian meal per week. I am not trying to convert you to a vegetarian. This suggestion will simply encourage you to seek out new and interesting food and to cook in a new way. Also, vegetarian meals, when planned and prepared well, are very nutritious and are low in saturated fat, sugar, and other junk. This meal does not have to be gourmet. There are a lot of quick, convenient options.

Get your family involved and get them on your side. Let them know you're focusing on better health for the whole family. If you have a stubborn "meat and potatoes" family member, ask them to humor you. After all, it's for their own good.

Beyond that, simply begin to phase out the junk food and introduce the real food. Discuss with your family why their health is important and what you've read in this book. Spouses may or may not be willing participants, but children are sponges for knowledge and will soak up the information. Keep reminding them how bad food will harm them and how much our bodies need the good food. And the bottom line is, you are in control. If you don't buy the junk, it will not be available to them at home. Pull rank if you have to!

Your New Grocery List

Following are some ideas for healthier choices you can make at the grocery store. Some of these items can only be found at a health food store, but if enough of us change our lifestyle, that can change.

Organic Dairy Products	Milk, half & half, butter, sour cream, cream cheese, cheese, etc.
Soy Milk	Soy milk can be found in most grocery stores.It used to have a reputation for tasting funny or leaving an after taste. But, in recent years they have really improved on this product. You can buy soy milk enriched with calcium and vitamins. A serving of enriched soy milk has the same calcium and vitamin D as a serving of cow's milk. You can cook with it; you may have to experiment with the consistency. Plus, soy milk is loaded with a lot more health benefits. It comes in different flavors and in the form

of protein shakes, energy shakes, etc. (I love Silk Chocolate Soy Milk by White Wave.) Also, you can buy soy milk in individual serving boxes with straws for the kids. With all of the encouraging news out about the benefits of soy, this is a real winning alternative to dairy.

Rice Milk

Rice milk is a great substitute for cow's milk and is preferred over soy milk by some people. As with soy milk, you can buy rice milk enriched with calcium and vitamins, in different flavors, and in individual serving boxes. You can cook with it as well. Vanilla enriched rice milk is delicious on cereal. (I recommend Rice Dream by Imagine Foods the vanilla enriched and the chocolate are both delicious.)

Soy Cheese

At a health food store you'll find many interesting choices of non-dairy cheese products. I usually buy Veggie Slices (made with soy) by Galaxy Foods at my grocery store. Galaxy Foods has a wide variety of non-dairy food products and my grocery store carries a good selection. It is located near the produce section. Soy cheese comes in blocks, slices, and shredded. I love to make a grilled cheese sandwich with whole wheat bread, olive oil (instead of butter), and Veggie Slices. You can use soy cheeses to replace cheese in any recipe. They come in several different flavors. Galaxy Foods also makes cream cheese and sour cream, among other products. Try these or experiment with the brands and products you can find. They're really quite good.

Tofu

Don't be afraid of tofu! There's nothing weird about it. It is made from soy beans and is very healthy. Pick up a vegetarian cookbook, a block of tofu from your grocery store, and give it a try. Or you can buy it already prepared at a health food store.

Soy Butter
Olive Oil
Vegetable Oil
Canola Oil

I still use a little dairy butter from time to time,but I usually prefer Veggie Butter (also by Galaxy Foods) or other soy butter. If you were using margarine, I know you've thrown that out. You can replace it with organic dairy butter (most groery stores carry it), but don't go crazy. You still have to consider the saturated animal fat. Try spreading soy butter on your toast and muffins. Again, try different brands to find your favorite. For cooking, vegetable oils and canola oil are okay. Also, you'll want to introduce olive oil in to your diet. It can replace butter and other oils in your cooking and has many good health benefits. It contains antiox-idants and can help lower bad cholesterol. Plus, it's delicious.

Organic Eggs

Buy eggs from a source that does not use growth hormones or antibiotics on the chickens. Read the egg cartons. My grocery carries one brand of these type of eggs. Sometimes they're called "cage free" but make sure they're also "drug free".

Vegetarian "Meat" Alternatives

There are many companies that now offer meat substitutes in

many varieties. Morning Star Farms products can be found in the frozen foods section of most grocery stores. Their selections include: bacon, sausage, chic nuggets, chic patties, veggie hot dogs, veggie burgers, and more. Many other brands and choices can be found at a health food store. Sample different items to discover what you like. Many are delicious and very similar to the real thing. I'll caution you again to read labels. Some of these products may contain unwanted additives, but most are quite healthy. My children love the chic nuggets, which can be

prepared   in   the
microwave or oven.

**100% Whole
Wheat Bread**

This doesn't require a
lengthy   explanation.
Read labels and make
sure the first ingredient
is whole wheat. Beyond
that, try to find a brand
that does not contain
partially hydrogenated
oil. You may have to
shop a health food store.

Prepared, Packaged Food

Frozen Food & Mixes

For items such as frozen pizza, boxed macaroni and cheese, frozen waffles and pancake mix, look for the healthiest product you can find. My health food stores carry all of these. The healthier versions are made from natural ingredients, fewer additives, and no partially hydrogenated oil.

Snack Foods

Almost any snack food you eat can be replaced with a healthy alternative that is very similar. Search your grocery store (usually near the "diet" foods) for cookies, snack crackers, granola bars, and chips that are made from healthy (preferably organic) ingredients. If you can shop at a health food store you'll find a lot of good snack foods. Remember to read labels. Again, try different brands and selections to discover the good ones. But, don't overload! Even "healthy" junk food should be limited.

Desserts

As with snack foods, there are many good alternatives that taste similar to the sweet treats you crave. There are good ice cream treats made from soy and rice milk. And you'll find cookies, cakes, and pies made with healthier, organic ingredients. I have found that desserts are more difficult to find at grocery stores. But health food stores offer many choices. My family loves Tofutti non-dairy frozen dessert, by Tofutti Brands, Inc. It's made from tofu (soy). Rice Dream, by Imagine Foods, is a frozen dessert made from rice milk. It comes in many flavors and is quite delicious.

Beverages

Water, of course, should be your main beverage.But for something a little more exciting, try natural fruit juices, herb teas, flavored rice milk and flavored soy milk. You can find natural (no sugar added) juices in many delicious combinations. Or create your own. Herb teas are really popular now and are good hot or cold. Try sweetening them with honey. And experiment with the many varieties of rice and soy milk everages which range from beverages to chocolate to mocha and cappuccino. Also, there are many wonderful protein and energy shakes which are nutritious and heavenly.

Natural Sugar Substitutes

Honey, 100% Maple Syrup, Unrefined Sugar, Date Sugar, Stevia. Some of these can only be found at a health food store, including stevia. Stevia is relatively new on the scene. It is derived from a plant and is very

sweet. It comes in leaves,
liquid, and powder.

Chapter 5

In a Nutshell

Well, there you have it, my version of nutrition made easy. Hopefully you have learned some things and are ready and willing to make some changes. I believe that I have taken a whole lot of overwhelming information and made it readable and understandable. I know it can still be intimidating, even condensed and simplified. There are still so many things to consider and remember. But I know you'll be fine if you just take my advice and go slowly.

My goal with this book is to connect with people who would be considered beginners when it comes to healthy eating. I believe the vast majority of people will take steps to improve their diet and health if given a little help. And that's what this book is all about.

I wish we could all meet individually and swap ideas. I actually have started doing just that in my area. I have implemented nutrition workshops for parents at nearby schools and will soon expand to other groups. I am also going to start giving in-home workshops. People have been very receptive to my ideas, which reinforces my belief that people have good intentions and want to eat right, they just don't always know where to begin.

I decided to write this book and share this great information with other people to help them change their lives. Doing workshops is another way I can connect with people on a more personal level and help them. Now that you have the information, you can do the same. By simply discussing this book with others, or by giving them their own copy, you can help spread the word about good nutrition. Maybe you'll even want to hold nutrition workshops in your area. It doesn't matter how we share the knowledge, only that we **do** share it.

The best way to get other people to listen to you is to lead by example. When others see you looking and feeling better, they'll want to know your secret. When people notice that you're making healthier choices and feeding your family better, they'll want to know how to start and what to do. All you have to do is be ready with the information. What a tremendous difference we can make, one person at a time!

Bibliography

Appleton, Nancy. *Lick the Sugar Habit*. Santa Monica, Ca.: Choice Publishing Co., 1985.

Bishop, Gael. *The Importance of Hydration*. Healthy Living Guide website (April 11, 1999).

Carroll, David. *The Complete Book of Natural Foods*. New York: Summit Books, 1985.

Gordon, Jay. *Good Food Today, Great Kids Tomorrow*. Studio City, Ca.: Michael Wiese Productions, 1994.

Henner, Marilu. *Total Health Makeover*. New York: Harper Collins Publishers, Inc., 1998.

Hull, Janet Star. *Sweet Poison*. Far Hills, New Jersey: New Horizon Press, 1999.

Loiselle, Beth. *The Healing Power of Whole Foods*. Nicholasville, KY.: Healthways Nutrition, 1993.

Parachin, Victor. *365 Good Reasons to be a Vegetarian*. Garden City Park, New York: Avery Publishing Group, 1998.

Roel, Evelyn. *Whole Food Facts*. Rochester, Vermont: Healing Arts Press, 1988.

Subramuniyaswami, Sivaya. "Discussing Vegetarianism with a Meat Eater: a Hindu View." Himalayan Academy website (April 1999): 1–19.

Weil, Andrew. *8 Weeks to Optimum Health*. New York: Alfred A. Knopf, Inc., 1997.

"Bottled Water and Your Teeth." *Self Healing* (February 1999): 8.

"On Fitness: Savoring Soy-From Little Beans Many Benefits Grow." *Seattle Times* (January 28, 1996).

"10 Reasons to Eat Soy Foods." *Healthy Living Guide website* (April 11, 1999).

"Water." *Healthy Living Guide website* (April 11, 1999).